50 natural ways to
better sleep

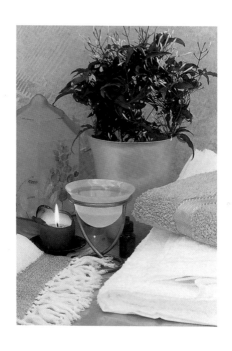

50 natural ways to
better sleep

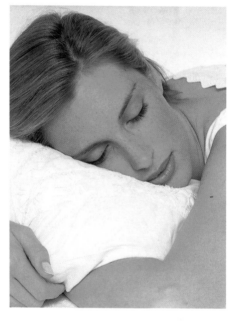

Tracey Kelly

LORENZ BOOKS

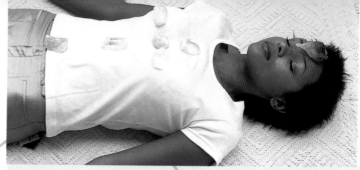

contents

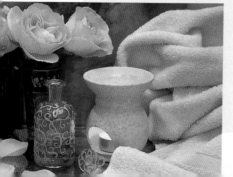

50 natural ways to...

better sleep

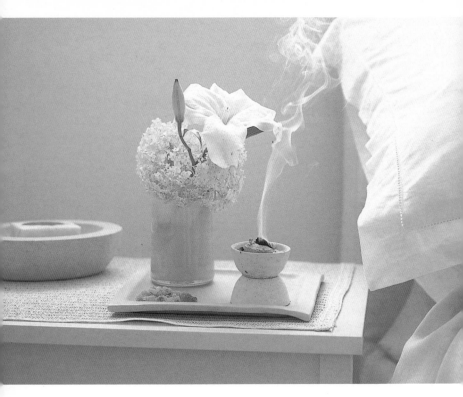

introduction

The average adult spends between seven and nine hours asleep each night. We know that during this time, the body makes any necessary repairs. Toxins are eliminated, tissues and cells are rebuilt. The mind processes stress that has accumulated during the waking hours, reducing its adverse effect on the system. But even with extensive research in the laboratory, many of the functions of sleep remain a mystery. One thing is certain, though – without it, the body and mind cannot operate properly. If sleep is missed or of poor quality for long periods of time, both our physical and mental health suffer. Sleep deprivation takes its toll on your productivity, your enjoyment of life and your looks.

Fortunately, there are many effective ways to stave off temporary bouts of insomnia and ensure continual deep sleep, night after night, allowing you to work and play at optimum energy levels.

exercise to relax

Keeping the body moving is essential for good sleep – without exercise, you will not be physically tired enough to rest at night. Aerobic activities such as

◄ A bedroom that is calm and peaceful will help you to relax at bedtime.

walking and cycling exercise the heart and tone the muscles, while some specific yoga techniques provide an excellent way to stretch and relax.

balance and perspective

At certain times, insomnia may result from stress. Massage techniques can ease tense necks, aching shoulders and uptight torsos, and face massage can be an instant calmer.

Some stress is an inevitable part of life, but when you need to achieve a state of inner calm, a range of meditation and visualization techniques can help you work through your insecurities, worries and anxieties. With practice, stress can be diminished so that it is no longer a cause of sleepless nights.

a calm environment

Lack of sleep can also be exacerbated by external factors such as noise, a "busy" atmosphere in the bedroom, or simply the wrong type of mattress. By making the best of your physical environment, you can reduce or remove many of these detrimental factors.

Following the principles of feng shui you can arrange your bedroom space to best effect and remove clutter that can clog free-flowing "chi" or energy. Choosing a calming room decor and lighting scheme can soothe the senses, while establishing a bedtime ritual can make sleep a pleasant and comforting experience to look forward to.

pampering treatments

In view of the many demands made by daily life, it is essential to find time to switch off from cares and worries in the evening, and indulge in some personal quality time. However busy you are, you should take time to wind down before trying to go to sleep, otherwise your mind will still be buzzing with the concerns of the day. Surrounding yourself with gentle

▼ A massage from your partner will help to ensure a good night's sleep.

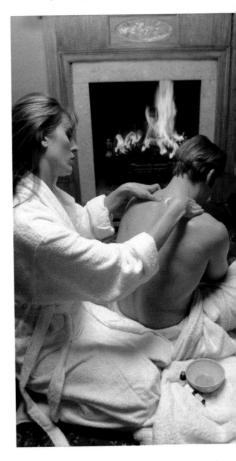

candlelight and sinking into a hot bath laced with aromatherapy oils or herbal sachets can go a long way to soothe and prepare your body for sleep. Essential oils such as lavender and clary sage added to the water help to diminish tension headaches and muscular aches, while bath bags or bath salts made with chamomile help to ease stress. You can also use the natural energies from flowers and herbs as a base for warming foot baths, soporific sleep pillows and effective sleep tinctures.

bedtime snacks

You ate dinner at 6pm; it's now 11:30pm and you're ready to go to bed, but now you're feeling hungry and thirsty again. What do you do? Instead of raiding the refrigerator for a substantial and perhaps indigestible

▾ A cup of fragrant chamomile tea at bedtime will help you drift off to sleep.

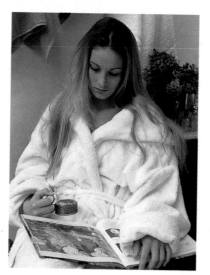

meal, it is better to opt for a light snack, such as toast with a topping, and perhaps a hot, comforting beverage. Try to avoid tea and coffee as they are stimulants and will tend to keep you awake if you drink them late in the day. Instead, herbal teas prepared for their sedative properties may be sipped in the evening, while warm, milky drinks are ideal for consumption before bed – milk contains peptides that calm the system. The occasional hot toddy can also provide a delicious way to wind down, and this is particularly good on a cold winter's evening, especially if you are suffering from a cold.

calming the psyche

Sometimes it is difficult to sleep due to excessive emotions, such as fear, excitement or anxiety. Crystal therapy can help to calm heartache; choosing the right stones can also calm restlessness and anxiety, and help to regulate sleep patterns. Crystals can be helpful when bad dreams and nightmares are keeping you awake, as can techniques such as visualizing a guardian angel or spiritual protector. When you have perplexing or mystifying dreams, it can be very helpful to write down what happened before you forget, so that you can ponder and try to analyse them later on. Working towards an understanding of your dreams adds an enjoyable richness to what can be the fascinating pageant of sleep.

▸ Make bathtime special with soft candlelight and fragrant oils.

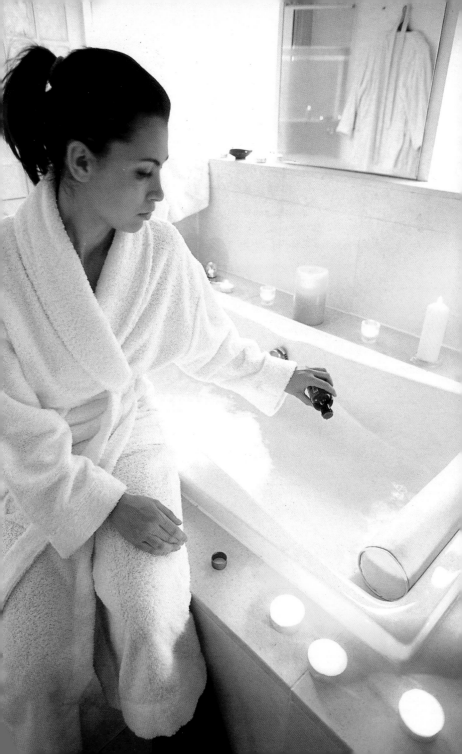

sleep treatments

This book is divided into sections that address different ways to achieve healthy sleep using natural remedies and techniques. It is designed so that you can select from many options to aid a state of rest, from relaxation techniques and aromatherapy baths, to creating the right bed-room atmosphere, to meditation and dream work.

To keep your body supple and relaxed, massage, reflexology and yoga techniques are suggested. A section on aromatherapy explores ways to relieve tension and irritation, and to rid the system of damaging anger and stress, while recipes for bath salts, sleep pillows and herbal teas are designed to soothe you to sleep.

Finally, esoteric sleep aids and quick fixes – from healing and calming crystals, to techniques for exploring and understanding your dreams – help to bring calm and balance to your sleeping and waking life. And if all else fails, try instant cures, such as sniffing an onion – which just might work.

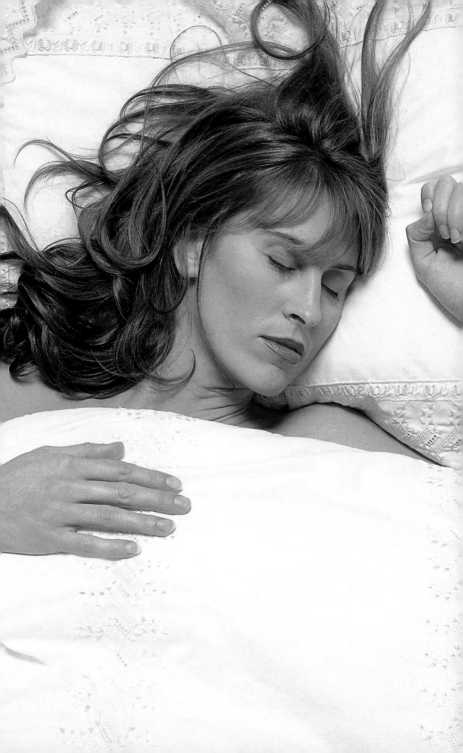

1

head & face relaxer

Headaches may be due to many causes – anxiety, sinus congestion or computer overuse – and can be a real deterrent to sleep. Simple massage strokes alleviate tension and promote relaxation.

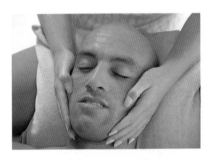

1 You may wish to use a little almond or grapeseed oil, rubbed into the hands, to smooth the movements. Using small, circular movements with all four fingers together, work steadily down from the forehead, around the temples and over the cheeks. Work slowly to ease tensions out of all the facial muscles.

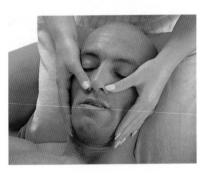

2 Press gently around the eye sockets, beginning near the nose. Smooth firmly around the arc of each socket beneath the brow bone, then glide firmly down to the nostrils and out towards the cheekbones. Next, move out to the jawline. Slide both hands under the cheekbones, softening the pressure at the sides of the face.

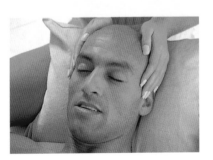

3 Draw the hands smoothly up the cheeks to the temples. Relax the hands and sweep the palms soothingly up over the side of the temples and scalp, then draw them away from the head.

2 tense neck easer

When you are fatigued, aching, tense muscles in the neck and shoulders make it difficult to get comfortable in bed. Use these self-massage techniques to target problem areas for fast relief.

1 Start by shrugging your shoulders then letting them relax completely a few times. Firmly grip your opposite shoulder with your hand and use a squeezing motion to loosen tension. Repeat on the other shoulder. This kneading action removes waste matter from tired muscles and moves fresh, oxygenated blood into them.

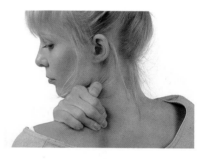

2 With the fingers of both hands, grip the back of the neck and squeeze in a circular motion to relax the muscles leading up either side of the neck. Work up to the base of the skull and down again to the shoulders.

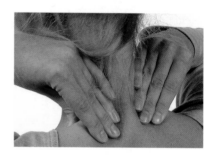

3 Move the thumbs in a circular movement across the neck and right up to the base of the skull. You should feel the bone as you apply moderate pressure. Rest for a few moments before standing and moving.

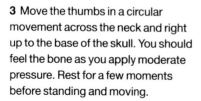
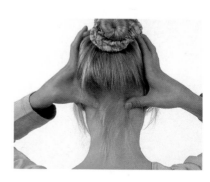

3 daily exercise

Some kind of physical exercise during the day is essential for a good night's sleep. Humans are designed to move – it is no use expecting to sleep easily and deeply if your body isn't tired.

Making time for exercise is of the utmost importance for a healthy lifestyle. Many people in sedentary occupations feel that they have no time for exercise, or are too tired at the end of the day. Exercise not only boosts physical stamina, but it also enhances your mental outlook and self esteem, through the release of endorphins, hormones that foster a positive mood. It also builds muscle tissue, and as you grow in physical strength, you will also feel stronger mentally and emotionally.

Spend as much time as possible outdoors, as sunlight helps to regulate the body clock. This is especially important during the short days of winter, when natural light will help to keep depression and SAD (Seasonal Affective Disorder) at bay.

Walking can be done almost anywhere, and it helps to keep the heart and other organs healthy. Activities such as swimming, tennis, squash, weight-lifting and dancing require more thought and planning, but they offer tremendous rewards and are very enjoyable. Whichever activity you choose, aim to exercise for at least 45 minutes three times a week – but for optimum fitness and to ensure restful sleep, try to make time for some exercise every day.

◀ *Jogging gets you out in the sun and fresh air, as well as exercising the lungs and heart.*

To relieve tension and

enhance restfulness

before retiring to bed, massage

the web between your thumb

and index finger on both hands.

5 yoga stressbuster

Used to calm the body and channel the mind, yoga is an excellent way to de-stress. The following technique focuses the mind on relaxing every part of the body.

Lie on your back with a bolster of blankets arranged under your upper body so that your shoulders are slightly elevated; this "opens" your upper chest and your lungs to allow free breathing (this is called the Savasana position). Spend a few minutes relaxing the body. Release tension from the feet and hands, the abdomen and face.

Calm your thoughts as you focus your mind on each part of your upper body in turn. Keep the eyes still and let the eyeballs relax down into the eye sockets. Relax the temples and forehead. Relax the bridge of the nose. Relax the cheeks by releasing them away from the eyes, then the jaws, moving the lower jaw a little way from the upper without tensing it.

Feel the connection between the ear passages and the jaws, and relax them. Keep the tongue still, letting it rest on the lower palate; allow the root of the tongue to recede into the throat, keeping the teeth lightly parted.

Next, relax your neck and throat by pressing the shoulders down and moving the shoulder blades into the back ribs. At the same time, bring the chin slightly down towards the throat. Quiet the vibrations of your vocal cords. End your relaxation here. Before getting up, turn on to your right side, with knees close to the chest and remain resting there for a moment or two.

▾ *Follow a simple yoga relaxation routine to unwind completely after a busy day.*

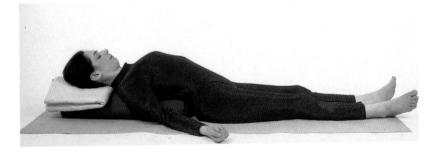

6 sensual massage

By learning basic massage strokes, you and your partner can touch each other with tenderness, sensuality and playfulness, relaxing each other's body and mind, enhancing the ability to sleep.

1 Begin by making sure the place you are going to massage your partner is warm and comfortable. With your partner lying on their front, sit at the top of their body. Put some oil in your hands, then place them on either side of the spine, and glide down the back. Move out to the sides and up the back again; repeat several times.

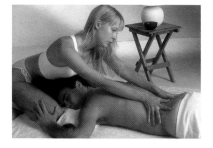

2 With a gentle motion, stroke down the centre of the back, with one hand following the other smoothly, as if you were stroking a cat. As one hand lifts off the small of the back, start again with the other at the neck. Continue this movement for several mintues.

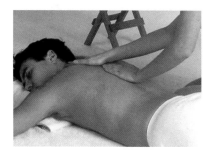

3 Place both hands on the upper back and stroke outwards in a fan shape. Work down the back and buttocks, using the fanning action.

CREATING THE AMBIENCE
See that the room is well-ventilated, and the lighting soft and soothing, perhaps using candles.

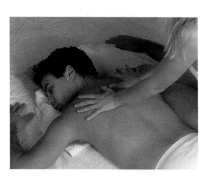

7

body & mind balancing

Learning to relax is crucial for maintaining a healthy body and mind. By letting go of tension, you will achieve a state of balance that allows easy and satisfying sleep, night after night.

Along with a nutritious diet, an exercise programme and a positive attitude, relaxation will help you keep your balance and perspective, even at those times when being under pressure is unavoidable. It can be beneficial to do the following exercise in the early evening, when you come home from your job or have finished your chores for the day. You can also use this technique to give yourself a midday oasis of serenity, if you can find a quiet place to stretch out for ten minutes. Deep, steady breathing will oxygenate your bloodstream, relieving stress on all the organs, including the brain, thus helping the thinking processes.

whole body relaxation
Lie down in a straight line, with shoulders relaxed and aligned on the floor. The arms should be straight – but not rigid – with elbows alongside the waist, palms turned upwards. Relax your head and close your eyes. Breathe in deeply down to your diaphragm (lower abdomen), and allow your body to sink into the floor. Breathe out slowly and relax. Focus attention on your breathing: listen as you inhale and exhale, and notice how quiet your deep breathing can become.

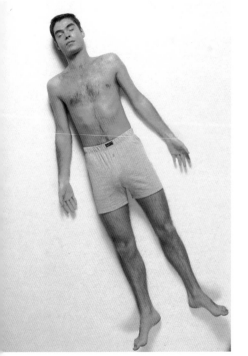

◄ *A daily ten-minute period of relaxation relieves stress and helps clear the mind.*

8 meditative visualization

Meditating can help bring mind and body into a state of harmony. It is a way to balance an active life with calming periods of inner reflection, and has the benefit of promoting easy, restful sleep.

Regular meditation, combined with positive affirmations, can help you to "centre" your mind, alleviating stress and allowing you to see a clear way forward through the daily problems and challenges you may face.

ease into meditation

Choose a quiet place for meditating, one where you won't be interrupted. Get into a comfortable position: sitting cross-legged is a traditional pose, but you may sit in a comfortable chair. Close your eyes, breathe deeply with your hands resting on your lap, and allow all thoughts to slowly leave your mind, as sand trickles through the neck of an hourglass. You may wish to focus on a word, or mantra, such as "OM": repeat this over and over until tension has left your body and mind. Or you could visualize a colour, allowing it to surround and suffuse you with its calming rays.

Allow 10 to 20 minutes each time you meditate; doing this twice daily is an effective way to restore composure. Informal meditation can be done any time you need a break; close your eyes for a few minutes and breathe deeply.

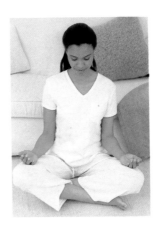

▲ Before you begin meditating, make sure that you are relaxed and comfortable.

AFFIRMATIONS

Speak or read these affirmations each night when you go to bed to remind yourself of your inner strengths before going to sleep.

- I enjoyed solving the problems I dealt with today, having done the best I could do.
- I enjoyed being calm and patient today, even when others were not.
- I will sleep deeply and peacefully, to awake in the morning fresh and full of energy.

9 leaving troubles behind

This meditation is sometimes called the "railway tunnel". Designed to help you focus on the present and leave you unfettered by past worries, it can be a very effective means of paving the way to sleep.

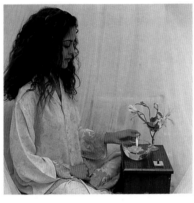

◀ To help focus your mind, light a candle before you begin the meditation.

Imagine strolling along a path between two high banks, with a dull, cloudy sky above ... a heavy back-pack makes your steps heavy and slow. ... You trudge along, feeling damp and cold. You reach the entrance to an old railway tunnel ... It is very dark, but you can see a point of light at the end, which is reassuring.... As you enter, all your self-doubts begin to surface ... you are aware of your failings and regrets.... Let them rise gently to the surface of your mind. The back-pack is getting lighter as they surface.

There is a pool of light on the floor ahead from an air shaft. As you go through the light, you remember a happy time, when you felt really good about yourself. As you move into the darkness again, you feel lighter; your back-pack is emptying, but the doubts are rising to the surface once more.... The circle of light at the end of the tunnel is growing, but here is another air shaft. As you pass through the light, another good memory comes into your mind. Now you are back in the gloom, but it doesn't seem as intense as before. It is getting lighter and warmer, and you experience more good memories.... As you near the end, you notice that the sun has come out, and you feel as if your load has disappeared. Warmth begins to replace the cold you felt before.

Eventually, you step out into the sunshine with a light tread, valuing yourself and the world much more. You realize you have so many opportunities awaiting you, and new chances to accomplish things. Your contribution is important, and you are a valuable and lovable person.

10 steps to sleep

The following visualization is similar to the traditional sleep cure of "counting sheep". Try taking a few deep breaths before beginning, as you prepare to let go of the day's cares.

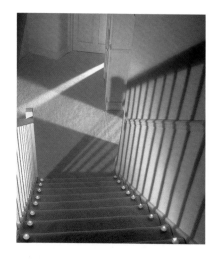

◄ *Visualize a staircase, inviting you down into a state of complete relaxation.*

stairway visualization

Imagine taking the first steps down, relaxing and letting go, feeling beautifully at ease and at peace. On step 8, you are becoming more relaxed ... on step 7, you are drifting deeper ... and deeper ... down still.

By step 6, you are calmer ... and calmer.... Halfway down, you are letting go and feeling good. On step 4, you are relaxing even more ... By step 3, you are sinking deeper.

On step 2, you are enjoying pleasant, peaceful feelings, half-awake, half-asleep. On step 1, you are feeling beautifully relaxed. On reaching the the bottom, you are so pleasantly relaxed, you can allow your mind to drift into sleep....

Imagine a staircase stretching down in front of you, made up of ten steps covered in soft, natural-coloured carpet, perhaps lit with candles or lanterns.You are standing on the tenth step. Count backwards from 10 to 0, and as you count backwards, imagine each number as a step, and each step as a step down the staircase into deeper and deeper levels of relaxation, so that by the time you get to 0, you can allow yourself to be as deeply relaxed as you can manage, while still being aware of the sounds around you.

VISUALIZATION TIPS
• Make sure you are warm and comfortable before you begin.
• If distracting thoughts enter your mind during the visualization, just let them drift on out.

11 instant relaxation

Once you begin to experience the positive effects of meditation, you can utilize "triggers" – evocative words and images that take you back into a state of relaxation – during the day or to aid sleep.

If you have imagined being in a certain place, or speaking a certain word or phrase during meditation, you can do so again to evoke the same positive feelings. For example, you may have imagined yourself sitting near a peaceful lake: if you conjure up that image again during a stressful meeting or a traffic jam, the memory will help you to relax instantly.

Repeating words or catch-phrases that mean much to you – such as "field of flowers" or "entering the dream" – can have the same calming effect, and will bring an instant pause to stress. If you are lying in bed, restless, be patient and pursue the image or word until you are enveloped in a sense of calm.

trigger happy
You may be aware of certain physical symptoms during meditation, such as a tingling sensation in the hands or feet: this can be a useful trigger, too. Imagine that you feel those symptoms, and within seconds you will gain the feelings associated with meditation. This can be especially useful before an important meeting, or on any occasion

about which you may be feeling a little apprehensive.

Use the triggers to gain the calm confidence you need and to put things into their proper perspective. With practice, your mind will accept the linkages you have created, and will respond to these signals at any time, quickly and easily, giving you instant access to all the benefits that come with deep contemplation.

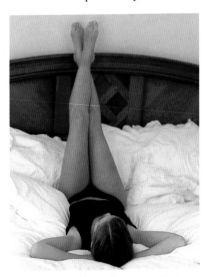

▲ Use the triggers acquired in meditation to achieve calm whenever you need it.

When future tasks are

keeping you awake at night,

free your mind by

writing a "to do" list

of things you need to

accomplish tomorrow.

13

the serene bedroom

The bedroom is one of the most important rooms in the house. The Chinese principles of feng shui can help you to arrange it so that the room is suitable for relaxing, regeneration and romance.

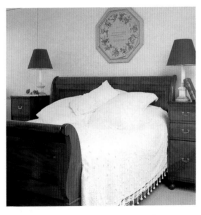

We spend about a third of our lives in bed, so it is fundamental to make the bedroom peaceful and relaxed. Feng shui governs the placing of furniture and objects so that "chi", or energy, can flow in the most propitious way. It enhances a serene environment.

The best position for the bed is diagonally opposite the door, so that you can see who is entering the room. If a line of chi between the door and a window crosses the bed, it is thought to cause illness.

Keep electrical equipment out of the bedroom completely, as it detracts from the main function of the room.

◄ *Ideally, mattresses should be raised off the floor and made from natural materials.*

Harmful electromagnetic waves – even from clock radios – can have an adverse effect on sleep.

Overall symmetry is important: side tables should complement each other's positions, and pictures should be hung in pairs. Photographs of parents, children and friends should have no place in a couple's private space. Mirrors in the bedroom should not face the bed. The Chinese believe that the soul leaves the body when we sleep and will become disconcerted if it comes across itself in a mirror.

CLEARING CLUTTER

Clear unnecessary clutter from the bedroom to create a sense of calm and enhance the flow of chi:
- Medicine bottles
- Cosmetics
- Used tissues
- Piles of clothes
- Old unworn clothes and shoes
- Full waste bins
- Work and papers
- TVs and music systems

14 a relaxing space

The physical set-up of the bedroom can go a long way towards helping you wind down at the end of the day. From lighting schemes to mattresses, you can facilitate maximum relaxation.

▸ *Use soft lighting beside your bed rather than harsh overhead lights.*

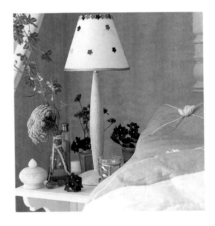

The most important item of furniture in the bedroom is the bed itself: a comfortable, supportive mattress is essential for restorative sleep. Shop around carefully for one that suits your weight and build. If a mattress is too soft or too firm, not only might it prevent peaceful slumber, it may be bad for your back as well. The surface should support your spine but give slightly. If you buy a mattress and find – after a trial week or two – that you've made a mistake, it is best to give in and buy another.

clouds of colour

Swathing your room in peaceful colours such as ivory, sky blue or delicate rose can have a wonderfully calming effect on the nervous system. Soft furnishings such as curtains and bedlinen should be soft, luxurious and tactile. Use only natural materials, they last longer than synthetics and "breathe" more easily.

Choose a lighting scheme that optimizes rest. Veto harsh, overhead lights in favour of small lamps. Try amber or soft-light bulbs of low wattage, keeping a brighter directional lamp at your bedside for reading. Candles are very soothing and can aid meditation and winding down, but remember to blow them out before you go to sleep.

RELAXATION TIPS
• Don't keep computers or work in the bedroom, as you will be unable to forget the cares of the day.
• Read a relaxing book. A tense thriller may keep you awake.

15 soothing bedtime ritual

As you approach bedtime, carrying out a familiar ritual – one on which you needn't spend much thought – is part of the process of shifting gears down towards sleep.

Many people find that a bedtime routine – such as taking a leisurely bath, preparing a hot drink and reading poetry – makes bedtime comforting and familiar. If you have children, your own rituals will be even more precious as a method of easing into slumber once you have said goodnight to them. This is your own time to enjoy peace and privacy.

Once you have decided to turn in for the night, unwelcome intrusions from other housemates or family members can be deterred by hanging

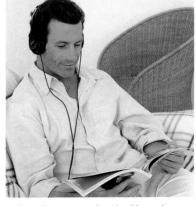

▲ If you listen to music at bedtime, choose something gentle and relaxing.

a "do not disturb" sign on the door. If friends often telephone late, don't bother taking the call – let the answering machine take them.

Music or your favourite late-night radio programme can ease your mind before sleep. If you like to read in bed, allow yourself time for it and go to bed earlier so you get as much sleep as you need. It can be comforting to keep favourite images or objects near your bed and glance at them before you sleep, to remind you of people you love and happy times.

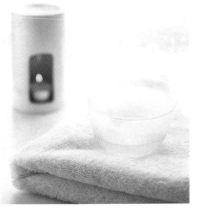

▲ Make a relaxing scented bath part of your regular evening routine.

16 tuning out the noise

Noise has an increasing presence in life, whether from neighbours, machines, dogs, road traffic or aircraft. But you have a right to a good night's sleep and there are ways to minimize the problem.

It is sometimes difficult enough to wind down before sleep, without noise augmenting the problem. In crowded cities, background noise can make life a misery and lead to insomnia and bad dreams – but you can take steps to tackle the problem.

peace and quiet

If you live on a busy road, or under a flight path, choose the room furthest away from the road or air route to be your bedroom. It may be worth investing in double-glazing. Terraced housing and poor flat conversions also present problems, as even the normal, everyday sounds of footsteps can echo through adjoining flats or houses. It is possible to install false walls or acoustic tiling – such as that used to soundproof recording studios – against party walls. This may seem an expensive move, but in the long term, a consistent lack of sleep will always be more expensive in terms of energy and quality of life lost.

noisy neighbours

If your neighbours are playing loud music, or hammering and drilling late at night, the first step is to have a word with them and come to a reasonable compromise – most people want to get on with their neighbours.

For very raucous parties where gentle reminders have been ignored, it may be necessary to inform the police, who will try to enforce some level of quiet. As a general rule, it is customary to keep noise to a friendly minimum between the hours of 11pm and 8am. Some people need reminding of this.

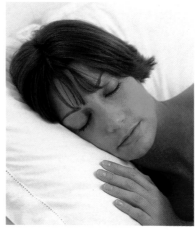

▲ Good-quality earplugs can help you to sleep undisturbed in a noisy environment.

17 sedating aromas

Using an oil burner to disperse essential oils is a wonderfully fragrant way to calm an overactive mind and lull your tired body to sleep. Some essential oils have a gentle sedative effect.

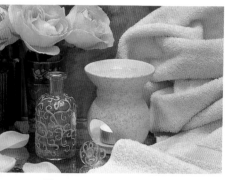

▲ Use rose essential oil to create an uplifting romantic atmosphere at bedtime.

Oil burners come in many styles, but they all heat essential oil in water so that it vaporizes as steam and can be inhaled. Most contain a candle or nightlight, and they should never be left unattended or around an unsupervised child, and should not be left burning overnight.

blending oils

Relaxing, restorative oils to alleviate depression and nervous tension include basil, bergamot, camphor, chamomile, clary sage, jasmine, lavender, neroli, rose, sandalwood, thyme and ylang-ylang. Chamomile,

juniper, lavender, marjoram, neroli, rose and sandalwood have a sedative effect. Cedarwood, juniper, melissa, neroli, peppermint and rose are calming and uplifting.

You can use the oils on their own or in a combination of two or three to create a serene atmosphere. Place 6–8 drops of oil in the filled water chamber of the burner. Add more water and oil if necessary.

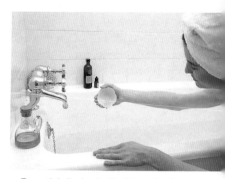

▲ Essential oil mixed with skin-softening almond oil can be added to the bath water.

> **STORAGE**
> Essential oils need to be kept in a cool place in airtight containers – dark glass bottles are best for long-term storage.

18

dispelling anger & anxiety

Negative feelings can leave you tossing and turning at night, instead of getting the rest you need. Aromatherapy oils can help dispel bad feelings before they cause sleepiness.

The ill effects of angry and anxious feelings can range from irritability and confusion, to impatience and explosive outbursts of rage. Coping with them is crucial for health.

dismantling anger

When allowed to fester, anger can certainly disturb sleep, so it is important to come to terms with the feeling and handle it in a positive, constructive way. Try to get to the root cause: why are you angry? Then think of ways to alleviate the feeling, i.e. expressing it calmly to another person. If you are angry with yourself over a mistake you may have made, remember that you are only human, and work on ways to rectify the situation that is troubling you.

diffusing anxiety

Stress and anxiety can be major factors in insomnia. Ongoing worries, perhaps over money or relationships, create tension that has a detrimental effect on your nervous system, outlook and sleeping patterns. If this anxious state continues, it can lead to illness.

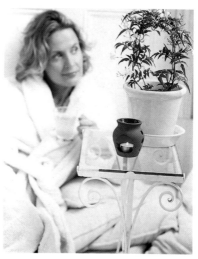

▲ Essential oils help to combat negativity and allow you to see things in perspective.

Regular exercise will help rid your system of the adrenalin produced by an anxious state, and meditation will help to restore your equilibrium. Relaxing essential oils – geranium, lavender and lemon – can help calm anger, while oils that are analgesic – basil, cedarwood, juniper and melissa – can help overcome fear and anxiety. Place a few drops in an oil burner or on a tissue and inhale the vapours.

To quell **feelings** of restlessness or irritation **at night,** place one or two drops of rose, **frankincense** or chamomile oil on to your **pillow.**

20 alleviating headaches and indigestion

Used in small amounts, pure essential oils can be added to hot tea to soothe away the stress of tension headaches and indigestion, thereby facilitating restful sleep.

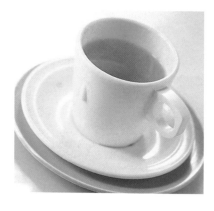

◄ If you find a cup of tea soothing, you can add to it the benefits of pure essential oils.

OIL TIPS
• Use only organic essential oils of therapeutic quality from a reputable source for adding to drinks.
• Absolutes or resins should never be ingested in this way.
• These methods should not be used for the treatment of children, but are suitable for the elderly.
• Never put essential oils directly into a drink, it will taste far too strong and will be very unpleasant.

To ease two common causes of restless sleep – headaches and stomach upset – pure essential oils can be added to a hot tea base. Choose oils that target the specific symptoms. For example, if you are suffering from indigestion, peppermint, fennel, chamomile and dill are all good choices. If your head is throbbing, lavender may ease the pain.

CAUTION
Do not increase the dosage without consulting a medical practitioner. The oils contain natural chemicals that are toxic in larger amounts.

making tea with oils
Tannin-free china or rooibos (red bush) tea make the best base for insomnia teas. Put 2–3 drops of essential oil on to the tea leaves or tea bag, add 1 litre/1¾ pints/4 cups of hot water, stir well, then remove the tea leaves or bag. The tea will taste best without milk.

Never pour essential oils directly into a cup of tea, as they will not disperse. Any tea that isn't drunk immediately may be stored in the refrigerator and reheated as required.

21 oils for insomnia

Not everyone needs an eight-hour quota of sleep, but if you find yourself awake night after night, perhaps due to a temporary problem or anxiety, aromatherapy oils may help.

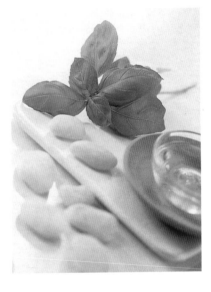

◀ *Essential oils with sedative properties are an ideal addition to your evening bath.*

- **Basil:** This oil calms the nervous system generally.
- **Chamomile:** A very calming and relaxing oil, and a good choice when indigestion hinders sleep.
- **Clary sage:** This has a sedative and almost euphoric action, but do not use if you have had alcohol – it can give you nightmares or a hangover.
- **Lavender:** Not only very soothing, but also analgesic, so if you have any aches and pains that lead to insomnia, this oil is probably the best remedy.
- **Marjoram:** In large amounts it is quite sedating – but it can leave you feeling groggy, so use sparingly.

People have different sleep patterns, but if you do find yourself unable to sleep, whatever your natural pattern, the following essential oils can help, especially when added to a very warm bath at bedtime. Just add 4–6 drops to the water and swirl to disperse. Do not use the same oils for more than two weeks at a time.

▶ *Add 1–2 drops of oil to hot water for a soothing steam inhalation or foot bath.*

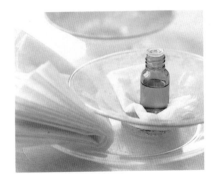

22 soothing massage oil

Aromatherapy essential oils can be combined with delicate carrier oils to help create a healing and comforting massage experience that can gently allow your body to wind down before bed.

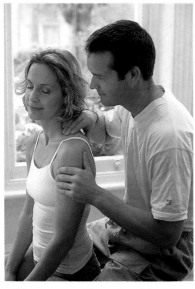

▲ The area around the neck and shoulders is particularly prone to holding tension.

A pleasant blend of lavender, clary sage and chamomile oils is ideal when you want to soothe away stress and help relieve feelings of nervous tension. Ideally, enjoy this oil as part of a full body massage, but when this is not possible, try gently massaging in a couple of drops of the oil behind the ears, using a circular motion.

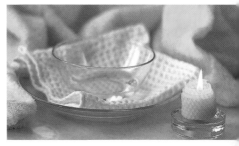

▲ Use a light carrier oil such as almond, and warm it gently in your hands before use.

tension-relieving massage oil
45ml/3 tbsp almond oil
1.5ml/¼ tsp wheatgerm oil
10 drops lavender, 5 drops clary sage,
    5 drops chamomile essential oil

Pour the almond and wheatgerm oils into a 50ml/2fl oz glass bottle, add the essential oils and gently shake to mix. Store in a cool, dark place.

CAUTION
Although generally safe, clary sage and chamomile oils should be avoided during pregnancy. If in doubt about any essential oils, consult a medical practitioner.

23 heavenly tubs

Being immersed in warm water is one of the most comforting sensations you can experience. For an antidote to a busy day, simply run a bedtime bath and enjoy the tranquillizing effects of water.

Many cultures throughout history have recognized the healing and health-giving properties of water, and spa resorts have been built around natural springs from ancient times to the present day. But you needn't be near a spa to enjoy water – a pampering and relaxing treat is only as far away as your own bathroom.

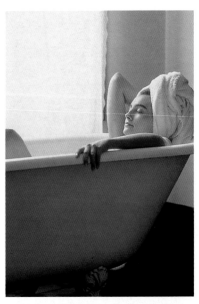

▲ *Think of the bath as a place to relax and unwind as much as a place to get clean.*

soothing waves
It is essential to find time to switch off from cares and worries. By reserving half an hour for yourself and locking the bathroom door, you can ensure a little oasis of peace while you read, listen to music or a play, or just lose yourself in pleasant contemplation – whatever you find most calming.

The ideal time for an evening bath is about an hour before going to sleep. This gives your body a chance to cool down slightly before you get into bed. Have big, fluffy towels on hand and a moisturizing cream or body oil to round off the sensual experience.

bathtime scenery
You can enhance your bathing pleasure by creating a room that cossets all your senses. Paint the room a watery colour, such as sea green or azure blue. If you like plants, surround the tub with moisture-loving ferns and scented plants such as jasmine or stephanotis. Soften lighting by fitting flattering amber, peach or pink lightbulbs, or use lanterns. Make sure the room is warm in winter, and well-ventilated in summer.

24 sedative bath bags

Cloth bags filled with herb blossoms make a subtle and gentle addition to your evening bath – the sedative properties of these therapeutic plants wil help to soothe you to sleep.

A sleep-inducing mixture of lime, chamomile and hop flowers is a perfect wind down to an early night.

soporific bath bags
eight 30 x 10cm/12 x 4in rectangles
    of loosely woven fabric
needle and thread
50g/2oz chamomile flowers
50g/2oz lime blossom
25g/1oz hop flowers
50g/2oz coarse oatmeal
lengths of ribbon or string

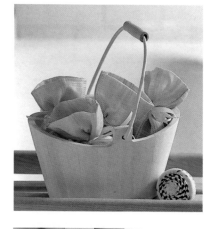

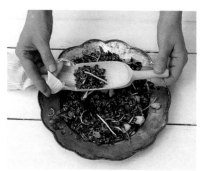

1 Fold the fabric rectangles in half and sew up three sides. Turn right-sides out. Combine the herbal ingredients and oatmeal and fill the bags with the mixture.

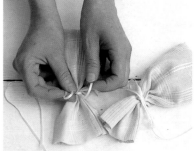

2 To finish, tie a large loop in a length of ribbon or string before using it to secure each bag. The loop can then be hung around the hot tap so that the running water flows through the bag. The materials make eight bags.

25 relaxing bath salts

A concoction of salts and aromatic flowers, herbs or oils can be added to the bath for a wonderful soak at bedtime. Although many salts are suitable, simple sea salt is used for this mixture.

Chamomile is a widely recognized sedative; for the following bath it has been combined with sweet marjoram, which is an effective treatment for insomnia.

These bath salts should be used only if you are planning to go straight to sleep after your bath: sweet marjoram is thought to be an anaphrodisiac, which means that it has the opposite effect of an aphrodisiac!

▾ *As well as having a sedative effect, the bath salts will heal and stimulate the skin.*

chamomile bath salts
500g/1¼lb/2½ cups coarse sea salt
10 drops chamomile essential oil
10 drops sweet marjoram essential oil
1–3 drops green or blue food
    colouring (optional)

Combine all the ingredients, mixing well with a wooden spoon, and pour into a glass jar with a lid. Place the lid on firmly and store in a cool place.

Add two heaped tablespoons of salts to the bath, pouring them under the hot tap as the water runs.

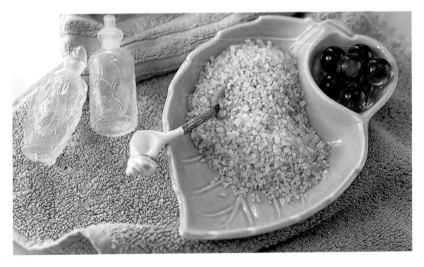

A few drops of lavender oil
added to your bath will
direct you towards slumber
in a sumptuous
cloud of scent.

27 easing herbal foot bath

Tired, sore feet can be a cause of wakefulness at night, especially if you have been standing or walking all day. A foot bath made with herbs is a soothing antidote that will help ease you to sleep.

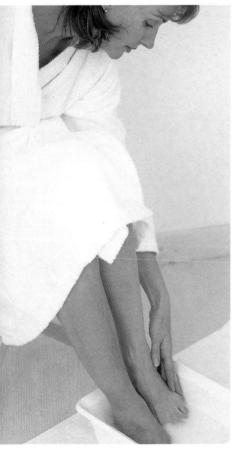

▲ A fragrant, soothing foot bath helps to warm and restore the whole body.

Peppermint is a particularly effective herb in foot baths. It has a cooling effect and helps to soothe aching muscles; rosemary is also useful for reducing pain. All the herbs listed will have a relaxing effect on the whole body as you inhale the fragrant steam rising from the hot water.

herbal foot bath for aching feet
50g/2oz mixed fresh herbs:
    peppermint, yarrow, pine needles,
    chamomile flowers, rosemary,
    houseleek
1 litre/1¾ pints/4 cups boiling water
15ml/1 tbsp borax
15ml/1 tbsp Epsom salts

Roughly chop all the fresh herbs, then place them in a bowl and pour the boiling water over them. Leave to stand for an hour. Strain the liquid, and add it to a bowl containing about 1.75 litres/3 pints/7½ cups hot water – the final temperature of the foot bath should be comfortably warm. Stir in the borax and the Epsom salts. Immerse the feet and soak them for about 15–20 minutes, then dry them thoroughly with a warm towel.

28 warming foot relaxer

A fragrant foot bath is ideal for refreshing tired feet. Not only does it comfort weary feet and calves, its warmth also relaxes the whole body and the scent of the herbs calms the mind.

The lavender in this mixture enhances feelings of serenity, and the lemon verbena restores balance to the nervous system.

lemon and lavender foot bath
15g/½oz dried lemon
    verbena leaves
30ml/2 tbsp dried lavender
30ml/2 tbsp cider vinegar
5 drops lavender essential oil

Place the lemon verbena and lavender in a basin and pour in enough hot water to cover the feet. When it has cooled to a comfortable temperature, add the cider vinegar and the lavender oil and swirl. Immerse the feet for 15–20 minutes, then dry well with a warm towel.

▾ A comforting herbal foot bath can also help to alleviate the symptoms of a cold.

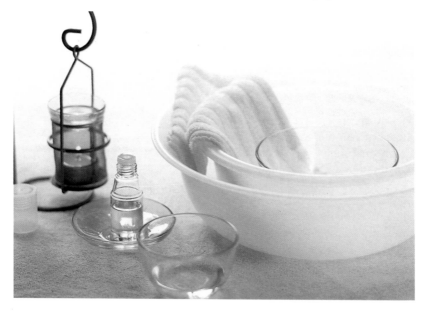

29 sleepy herbal pillow

A small pillow filled with calming herbs and flowers can help you to get to sleep at night. You will continue to benefit from its sedative effects all night, waking refreshed from untroubled sleep.

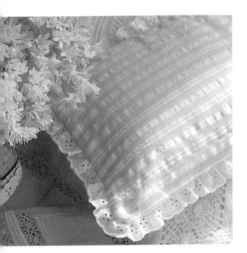

▲ Fill a small pillow with herbs so that you can benefit from their aroma as you sleep.

sleep potpourri
115g/4oz/2 cups dried hop flowers
115g/4oz/2 cups dried rose petals
50g/2oz/1 cup dried chamomile
    flowers
25g/1oz/½ cup each dried jasmine,
    orange blossom and lavender
10ml/2 tsp ground orris root
5ml/1 tsp frankincense powder
5–6 drops neroli essential oil

Mix the ingredients together. Place in an airtight container and leave in a warm, dry place for about ten days.

▼ Lavender is a useful sleep herb, lifting depression and alleviating stress.

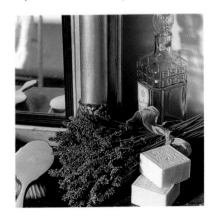

Prepare the potpourri first. All the ingredients for this are available from health food suppliers and herbalists. When the scents have combined and the potpourri is ready, make up a muslin (cheesecloth) bag and loosely fill it with the mixture. You can slip this bag into your ordinary pillowcase, or stitch a special small pillow and slip the herbal bag inside it. Tuck the pillow under your neck to enjoy its aroma as you go to sleep.

30 relaxing flower remedies

Bach flower remedies are vibrational essences. They work on the premise that natural energies can help redress emotional imbalances that may inhibit healthy functions such as sleep.

Developed by Dr Edward Bach in the early 20th century, Bach flower essences are sold individually or in mixtures designed to help alleviate specific complaints. The following remedies are prepared especially for sleep problems such as insomnia and nightmares. If you prefer, you can ask your health practitioner to create a tailor-made treatment for you.

fears and nightmares mix
This mixture is ideal for fears, night terrors and nightmares experienced by both adults and children. It contains a blend of Aspen, Cherry Plum, Mimulus, Rock Rose, Star of Bethlehem and White Chestnut.

insomnia mix
Used for releasing negative mental and emotional patterns, Insomnia mixture also works to soothe and quieten any excessive mental excitement that might prevent sleep. It contains Impatiens, Rock Rose, Vervain and White Chestnut.

morning glory
(*Ipomoea purpurea*)
This single flower essence can be useful if you are leading an erratic lifestyle. It works gently to support the body clock.

▼ *The absorption of the flower's energy in water is activated by the action of sunlight.*

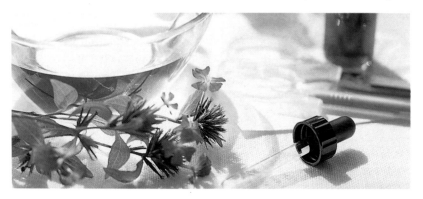

31 soothing lavender

The heady scent of lavender conjures up images of bountiful fields of blooms waving in the sunlight. But lavender has many uses: its healing and sedative qualities make it a key aid to natural sleep.

From ancient Egyptian times to the present day, lavender has been a star among medicinal plants. The Roman Pliny the Elder claimed that it was good for everything from dropsy to menstrual problems, and Elizabeth I drank lavender tea to cure migraines.

Lavender is still used in many herbal remedies. Cushions filled with dried lavender can help induce sleep,

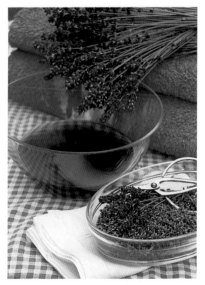

▲ *An infusion of fresh or dried lavender flowers has relaxing qualities.*

aid depression and alleviate stress; sniffing lavender oil sprinkled on a tissue has a similar effect. Fresh or dried flowers can be brewed into a tea that helps to cleanse the system and relieves headaches and stomach upsets. Lavender can also be made into a compress for external use to relieve sinus congestion, headaches, hangovers, tension and exhaustion.

If you are suffering from an evening headache or cold symptoms, or are feeling generally ill at ease, one of the following methods may help soothe you to sleep.

lavender infusion or tea
Pour boiling water into a cup, let it cool for 30 seconds, then add a teaspoonful of fresh or dried lavender. Cover the infusion and leave to steep for 10 minutes, stirring occasionally. Strain and drink the tea warm. Sweeten with a little honey if desired.

lavender compress
Soak a clean cloth in a hot infusion of lavender. Lie back and place the compress gently over your forehead, making sure not to get it in your eyes.

32 sleep-inducing violets

Tinctures are an effective way to extract the active medicinal constituents of plants. They keep well and may be taken when needed. This tincture uses sweet violets, which help to ease insomnia.

Tinctures are made by steeping the plant material in a mixture of water and alcohol. The alcohol draws out the active ingredients and also acts as a preservative. A 5ml/1 tsp dose of this remedy may be taken 3–4 times a day to relieve symptoms of insomnia and promote sound sleep.

sweet violet tincture
15g/½oz dried violet flowers
250ml/8fl oz/1 cup vodka
50ml/2fl oz/¼ cup water

1 Put the dried violet flowers into a glass jar, pour in the vodka and water then shake gently. The mixture will take on the a violet colour immediately.

2 Put a lid on the jar and leave in a cool, dark place for 7–10 days (no longer); shake occasionally. The tincture should darken.

3 Strain off the violets through a sieve lined with kitchen paper then pour the liquid into a sterilized glass bottle. Seal with a tight-fitting cork and store for future use in a cool, dark place. The tincture will keep for up to two years.

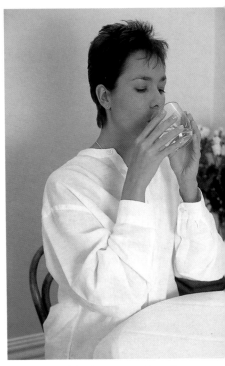

▲ You can add the tincture to a glass of water and sip slowly.

CAUTION
Never use industrial alcohol, or methylated or white spirits to make tinctures, as all these are highly toxic.

33 foods for restful sleep

You can help ensure sound sleep by eating from a variety of healthy foods throughout the course of the day. Avoiding foods that contain stimulants will also improve night-time rest.

bountiful sleep enhancers

Ensuring that your daytime diet is rich in B vitamins will help you sleep: the B group supports the nervous system and aids dream activity. Foods rich in Bs include green vegetables, nuts, seeds, eggs, seafood, soya, dairy foods and yeast extract.

Slow-burning carbohydrates such as oats, barley, rice and beans provide the body with a steady release of energy that helps keep the system on an even keel all day.

regulating the sleep cycle

Tryptophan is an amino acid found in turkey, milk, tuna fish and most carbohydrates. If there are sufficient levels of vitamin B6 in the body, tryptophan will aid in the production of neurotransmitters such as serotonin, which helps to regulates sleep patterns.

Calcium also helps release such serotonin. Choose foods such as broccoli, oats, sesame seeds, tahini and raw vegetables, rather than dairy products, which tend to increase mucus production. Kelp and other seaweeds are a rich source of calcium, as are watercress, dandelions and nettle.

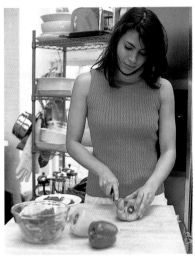

▲ Eat raw vegetables and unprocessed food throughout the day.

OVERSTIMULATING FOODS
It is best to avoid these substances
• **Caffeine:** this potent drug can make you edgy and irritable; avoid after 2–4pm.
• **Sugar:** refined sugars disturb metabolic processes; substitute honey, fruit sugars or maple syrup.
• **Chemical additives:** these are difficult for your body to process and may keep you awake.

34 perfect night-time food

Alhough doctors maintain that eating a large meal late at night is harmful to the system, hunger pangs can be a cause of wakefulness. A light snack provides the perfect solution.

When restlessness is due to a rumbling stomach, the best remedy is to treat yourself to a midnight snack. Stick to light foods – try wholemeal (wholewheat) crackers spread with a little peanut butter and a hot, milky drink. A small sandwich filled with turkey, avocado or cottage cheese is ideal, as these contain tryptophan, which may assist healthy sleep. Other easy-to-digest foods include a bowl of comforting oatmeal or a banana.

It is best to avoid foods that are difficult to digest, such as meats and high-fat content cheeses, or rich foods such as heavy sauces, pastries and cakes. Very sugary or acidic foods may give you heartburn, which will keep you awake. Always sit up for 15–20 minutes after eating before going back to bed, to give the food a chance to travel down the intestines.

drink up

Caffeine is best avoided from mid-afternoon onwards, but in general, hot drinks have a calming effect at bedtime, especially in cold weather. If you wake frequently in the night, a flask filled with a hot, caffeine-free

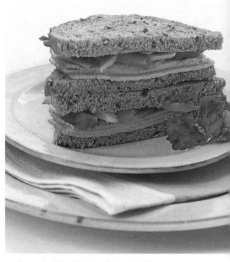

▲ A sandwich will calm late night hunger pangs, but pick an easily digestible filling.

drink such as herbal tea, chicory "coffee" or plain hot water can provide an instant soother. It also means that you needn't get up, thus making it easier to return to sleep.

If your wakefulness is due to sultry weather, iced chamomile or lemon balm tea will cool you down and provide instant relief.

35

herbs for peaceful sleep

If you often suffer from restless waking in the middle of the night, herbal remedies – taken either as a tea or tablet form, may help to quiet your nerves and settle an overactive system.

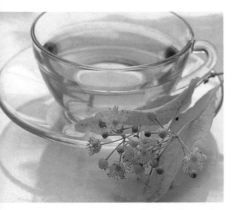

▲ Lime blossoms make a honey-scented tea that soothes nervous tension.

tranquillizing valerian

This herb is one of the most powerful sedatives in the plant pharmacopoeia. A tea made from valerian root has a rapid sedative effect, and it helps to ease nervous tension. When drunk after dinner and then directly before bed, it quickly alleviates symptoms of insomnia and facilitates sleep.

garden of sleepy herbs

One of the best bedtime herbs for those who have difficulty getting to sleep, chamomile has a soporific effect on the nervous system. It also gives relief to an overworked digestive tract, a common cause of insomnia. Another relaxing plant, lime blossom helps to calm nerves and reduce tension. Both of these herbs can be drunk as a tea: steep 5ml/1 tsp dried herb in a cup of hot water.

An ingredient in beer – and the cause of the pleasant sleepiness that a pint induces – hops is used for its restful effect. Wild lettuce has also been used to treat sleep problems, as have passionflower and lemon balm.

natural sleep cures

Sedative herbs are used in non-narcotic sleep tablets, which are taken once during the day and then an hour before bedtime. Valerian is usually the main ingredient – it may be used on its own or combined with hops, wild lettuce, lemon balm or passionflower.

> Dill seed acts gently to relieve colic – a common cause of wakefulness in babies and young children. Add 5ml/1 tsp lightly crushed dill seed to a cup of water and boil for 10 minutes. Strain well and allow to cool before drinking.

To help you sleep through the night, drink pleasant elderflower and lime blossom tea with a dash of nutmeg and a dollop of honey.

37 soothing tisanes

Made by steeping garden-fresh flowers in boiling water, tisanes provide a real treat for the taste buds. They can calm the nerves and send you to sleep on a proverbial carpet of blossoms.

The experience of drinking a tisane is a little like taking the garden's earthy energy into your system. The wonderful fragrances of these clean and clear tonics act as mood enhancers, and they are visually cheering – as well as tasting wonderfully

> Flower teas can be made from dried flowers when fresh blooms are not in season.

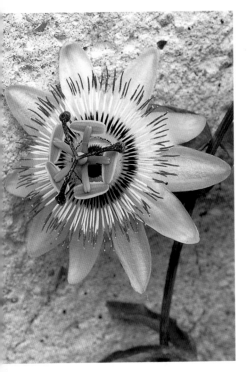

fresh. Many garden blossoms can be used for making tisanes, but the best ones for promoting sound sleep include: lavender, lime blossom, lemon verbena, dandelion, rosemary, rose petals, jasmine, peppermint, bergamot and passion flower.

passion flower tisane

The passion flower has wonderful sedative powers that are said to relieve nervous conditions such as palpitations and shakiness, thus helping to prevent insomnia.

To make a tisane, place one passion flower blossom (or 5ml/1 tsp dried passion flower) in a cup and add 250ml/8 fl oz/1 cup boiling water. Steep for 10 minutes, then remove the flower. You can drink a cup of this soothing tisane 3 times a day, and continue for 2–4 weeks.

◄ *For the best tisanes, cut passion flowers when the plant is producing its fruit.*

38 warming eggnog

This Scandinavian/American drink is usually
served cold, but this is a warm and creamy
version, guaranteed to soothe and relax on
a chilly autumn or winter's night.

Delicious eggnog is spicy and rich, so
a little goes a long way – a normal
serving is about the size of a small
wineglass. Drunk in the evening after
dinner, it provides an ideal way to
wind down before bedtime. The
drink can also be made without
alcohol – substitute 7.5ml/1½ tsp of
rum flavouring for the rum.

warming eggnog
serves 2
250ml/8fl oz/1 cup double (heavy)
   cream
1 long strip orange rind
1.5ml/¼ tsp freshly grated nutmeg
1 cinnamon stick
2 eggs, separated
30ml/2 tbsp caster (superfine) sugar
75ml/2½fl oz/⅓ cup golden rum
cinnamon sticks to serve

Warm the glasses. Pour the cream into
a small pan; add the orange rind,
nutmeg and cinnamon stick and
bring slowly to the boil. In a mixing
bowl, beat the egg yolks with the
sugar until really pale and creamy.
When the cream is boiling, pour on
to the egg mixture and whisk well.

Return the mixture to the pan and
stir over a very gentle heat until it
forms a custard as thick as pouring
cream. Do not overheat the mixture
or it will curdle. Warm the rum in
another pan. Stir it into the egg
custard, then whisk the egg whites
until soft peaks form, and fold them
into the hot custard. Serve in the
warm glasses, with a cinnamon stick.

▾ *Thick creamy eggnog, laced with rum, is
a delicious nightcap for a cold evening.*

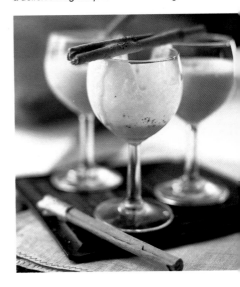

39 comforting hot drinks

When indulged in occasionally, a hot, alcoholic beverage can go a long way towards directing you to restful sleep. It is especially good when you are suffering from a cold.

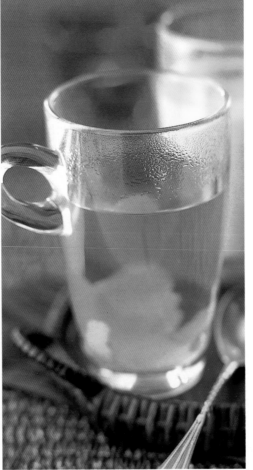

hot toddy

serves 2

2 strips lemon rind
4 slices fresh root ginger
5ml/1 tsp honey
175ml/6fl oz/¾ cup water
175ml/6fl oz/¾ cup
    whiskey or bourbon

Put the lemon rind, ginger, honey and water in a small pan and bring to the boil. Remove the pan and leave for 5 minutes. Stir in the alcohol and allow time for it to warm through. Rest a silver spoon in each pre-heated glass and strain in the warm toddy. Sip slowly.

CAUTION
As with all alcoholic beverages the sedative effect will be reversed if you consume too much alcohol.

◄ *A hot toddy will warm you up and relax tired muscles.*

40 sweet nutmeg milk

Milk contains substances that help restore feelings of calmness. When drunk at bedtime it can enhance restful sleep. The additions of honey and nutmeg give a soothing and tasty twist.

The first food that we consume as babies, milk has a soothing effect on the nervous system. It contains peptides that help to relieve stress and anxiety, and reduce nervous tension that can lead to insomnia. Many people find milk helpful in cases of indigestion – another common cause of wakefulness – particularly if it is sipped warm.

When drunk with honey and a sprinkling of nutmeg, a mug of warm milk makes a perfect bedtime nightcap. If you suffer from an allergy or sensitivity to dairy products, you can substitute goat, soya or oat milk for cow's milk.

hot nutmeg milk

This recipe makes one serving, but you can easily multiply the ingredients for two or more people. Heat 250ml/8fl oz/1 cup whole or semi-skimmed (low fat) milk in a milk pan, to just below the boiling point – do not scald. Remove from the heat and whisk until frothy. Stir in 10ml/2 tsp clear honey, then pour into a large mug and grate a light dusting of nutmeg over the milk.

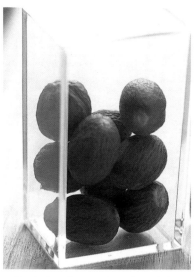

▲ For the best flavour, always buy whole nutmeg and grate it as you need it.

CAUTION
Use nutmeg sparingly. Although in small amounts its active ingredient, myristicin, enhances sleep and pleasant dreams, in large doses it is highly toxic. Just one to three grated nutmegs (in excess of 5ml/1tsp) can cause hallucinations, nausea and vomiting.

41

sleep pattern crystal cure

Sleeplessness can be brought on by a variety of causes. With the help of healing crystals, the situation can be overcome and your sleep patterns brought into balance once more.

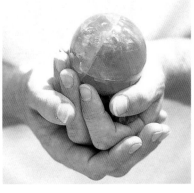

Different gemstones are said to ease various physical ailments, including disturbances in sleep patterns. The best way to use crystals is to get to know them by experimenting with them individually – one that works well for you may keep someone else awake. When you are half asleep and exhausted, the motivation to help yourself can be difficult to summon up. Having the right crystals at your bedside may help, so that you can simply pick one up without having to get out of bed.

▶ *Healing and calming, apple green chrysoprase encourages deep sleep.*

◀ *Holding an appropriate gemstone can help you relax and fall asleep.*

peaceful slumber

Chrysoprase has been found to encourage peaceful sleep. A tumbled stone can be put under your pillow, or on your bedside table.

When you are fearful, use a grounding and protecting stone such as tourmaline, staurolite, smoky quartz or tourmaline quartz and place it at the foot of your bed.

If tension and worry are causes of restlessness, amethyst, rose quartz or citrine may help. If your sleep pattern has been broken or disturbed by something you have eaten, a digestive calmer such as ametrine, moonstone or iron pyrites may be the solution.

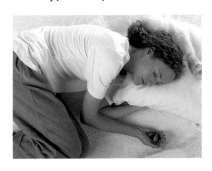

42 heart-healing crystals

There are many times in life when you may feel unhappy or heartsick, unable to do or say what you wish to. Healing crystals may help soothe the emotions so that you can sleep.

This layout of crystals is said to help calm an emotional upset and allow you to focus on a practical solution. As you work through it, you may notice signs of stress being relieved, including fluttering eyelids, deep sighs, twitching muscles, or yawning. Do not be alarmed if tearfulness results as aching feelings are released.

calming the heart

To clear emotional stress, you will need four clear quartz stones, a citrine, a small rose quartz and an amethyst. On the centre of the chest, place the rose quartz and surround it with four clear quartz points. If the points are placed facing outwards, they remove emotional imbalances. If they face inwards, they stabilize an over-emotional state. Just below the navel, place the citrine quartz with its point directed downwards, to increase a sense of security. Place the amethyst on the brow or above the top of the head to help calm the mind. If the release is too strong, remove the stones from the heart area and place a hand over the solar plexus.

▼ *Use this powerful crystal layout to help you cope when you are feeling unhappy.*

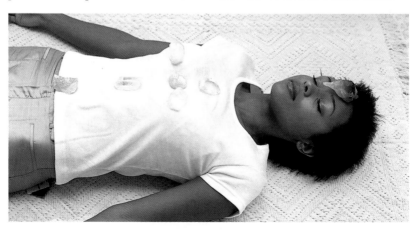

43 balancing & calming stones

After a hard day at work or with children, it can be difficult to wind down and relax. A simple placement of stones may help you to feel calm and refreshed after only a few minutes.

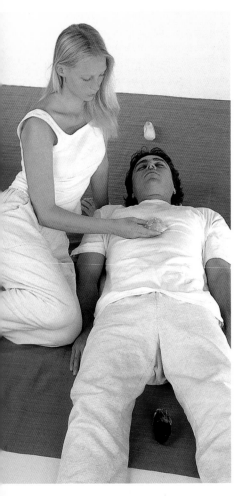

The three crystals used in this layout are all powerful healing stones and are useful in many situations. Clear quartz is said to quieten the mind and increase clarity, allowing you to neutralize the day's negative events, and put both positive and negative into perspective. Used pointing downwards, smoky quartz helps to release tension and re-establishes focus on the present moment, allowing you to take greater enjoyment in your leisure time. Rose quartz is said to balance the chakra system and the emotions.

balancing the system

Place a clear quartz crystal, with its point upwards, above the top of the head. Place a smoky quartz crystal, point downwards, close to the base of the spine (between the upper thighs or knees), then place a small rose quartz crystal on the centre of the chest. After 4–5 minutes, you should find that you feel refreshed and in tune with yourself again.

◄ *Lie down and relax completely to benefit from the calming influence of crystals.*

44 dealing with bad dreams

There are phases in everyone's life when they may be subject to bad dreams and nightmares. It is helpful to try to take a cool look at what these dreams might mean in the light of day.

Nightmares and fretful dreams often occur when life is in a state of upheaval. They may be due to anxiety about a current arrangement or the outcome of an upcoming event, or unresolved feelings or worries about yourself or other people.

The death of a loved one, illness, the end of a relationship, moving house, changing jobs, having a baby or getting married can all dredge up fears and anxieties. Even if a change is positive, it may produce anxious dreams that relay fears about your ability to "move with the times".

hidden obstacles

Sometimes bad dreams indicate the unconscious mind's attempt to bring hidden fears to the conscious mind, where they can be dealt with. In cases of long-term stress, bad dreams can bring the unresolved issues causing the problem to the surface. If you can make sense of your dream, you can try to apply what you've learned to your waking life.

Dreams can be an early warning system – they let you know when you need to reassess and de-stress. If

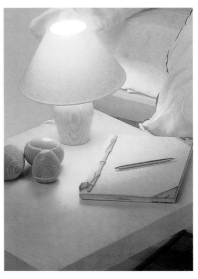

▲ If you write down your dreams, you will be able to ponder their meaning the next day.

you wake frightened or unnerved after a bad dream, turn on the light and assure yourself that you are awake and unharmed. It can be helpful to jot down the dream, thus "removing" it from your mind and on to the paper. If you have continual nightmares over a long period, you may wish to seek help from a therapist or counsellor to explore the underlining causes.

45

dream journal

Recording your dreams can give you valuable insights into the fabric of your dream life, tracing patterns that occur over time. It can also bring unconscious thoughts and needs into focus.

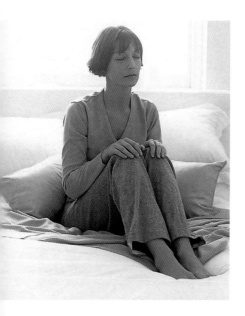

◄ *Work with your dream during the day, to try and bring it into focus and under control.*

Write down your dreams as soon as you wake, whether in the middle of the night, or first thing in the morning. Dreams have a very elusive quality and tend to slip away almost immediately, so it is best to capture them as soon as possible.

exploring the unknown

Use your journal to work with a dream when you are awake. You need to recall and replay it in a relaxed and conscious state, as being at ease makes your intuition flow more freely. Try sitting or lounging on the bed. Quiz the characters and places of the dream for answers to your questions: "Who are you? Why are you here? What are you trying to tell me?" Go with the first answers that pop into your mind, and try to apply them to your current situation; the dream's meaning should start to come into focus. Sometimes it takes a week or two of looking at a dream for its meaning to be digested and understood. The many books available on dream analysis and interpretation may help you explore dream symbolism further.

creative voice

Remember, dreams can be a vehicle for synthesizing ideas – people have been known to write great stories, compose beautiful music and solve scientific puzzles via their dreams, so recording them may lend inspiration for your future endeavours.

46

calling an angel protector

It can be very comforting to visualize a protective spirit or "guardian angel" before going to sleep. This could be any figure you feel will watch over you and keep you safe during the night.

Especially when you are feeling vulnerable, lonely, ill or troubled, it can be helpful to visualize the presence of someone who protects you as you sleep. This protector could be a traditional angel figure, or it could be a missed loved one such as a parent or grandparent. It could even be a strong animal – perhaps a bear or a cougar.

The following exercise will help you create a force field of light that surrounds you in your mind's eye, with your angel or protector nearby.

angelic light

While in bed, relax completely, lying flat on your back. Rest your arms at your sides and take a few deep breaths. Imagine a strong and powerful figure, one for whom you feel complete trust and friendship. Visualize your protector's features; talk to them, and feel their calming presence reassure you. You may want to point out anything that is particularly bothering you, and know

that your protector understands and wants what is best for you.

Now imagine your body surrounded by a pool of bluish-white light. The light envelopes you completely with its beauty and serenity. Let the light spread out to surround your bed, in pulsating waves of energy. Know that the protector watches over you and the light, guarding your sleeping self and keeping you from harm.

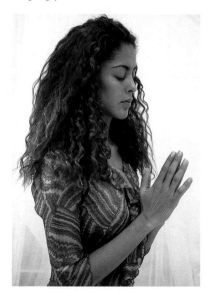

▸ *Call on your guardian angel before you go to bed to watch over you as you sleep.*

47 sleep cures

When slumber eludes you and you are left tossing and turning, it's time to rethink your bedtime tactics. Try adding one or more new practices to help you achieve a healthy night's sleep.

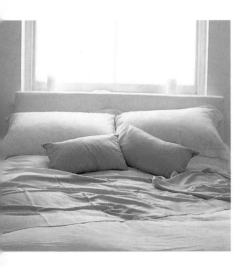

◄ *Try keeping your bed as a place for sleep only and rid the room of any distractions.*

can see fish swimming past.
• Visualize a boring scenario, such as a lecture you have no interest in.
• Read out loud the names and numbers from the phone book.
• Reserve your bedroom and the bed as a place for sleep only.
• Wiggle your toes gently until you fall asleep.
• Rub your stomach lightly.
• Cut up a mild onion, place in a jar by the bed and sniff before retiring.
• Think of ten wonderful things that have happened to you today.
• Squeeze all your muscles together tightly for a few minutes then relax.

instant fixes
If all else fails and you are still awake in the dead of night, try some, or all, of these quick cures.
• Lie on your back with your knees propped on a small pillow.
• Sleep with your head facing north.
• Get up at the same time every morning and go to bed at the same time every night for a week.
• Visualize yourself in a peaceful place, such as a field full of wildflowers with a gentle breeze blowing, or near a gently flowing stream where you

CAUTION
Avoid these sleep deterrents:
• Drinking excessive alcohol
• Smoking cigarettes
• Taking long naps in the afternoon
• Watching disturbing films or TV prior to bed
• Playing video games
• Listening to fast-paced or loud music

48 prayer for sleep

By reaching out to your god or the universe with a prayer before sleep, you will experience feelings of peaceful release and freedom from worry. Chanting can also help to set your mind at rest.

Many faiths have formal bedtime prayers – such as the Christian "Now I lay me down to sleep" – that are designed to comfort the individual and lend a feeling of protection during the seven or eight hours' absence from consciousness. This is a nice way to round off the day and complete your thoughts.

protection prayer
I ask God, the stars in the sky and the
    moon above
to look down upon me and all I love
to watch and protect us throughout
    the night
to keep us from danger and
fill our hearts and souls with golden
    light.

bedtime chant
Let me move beyond cares
Let me leave fear behind
Let me rest in a peaceful land
Let me wander to the farthest shores
    of dreams, to learn what I will and
    see what I see
then safely return when morning
    comes,
refreshed and ready for a new dawn.

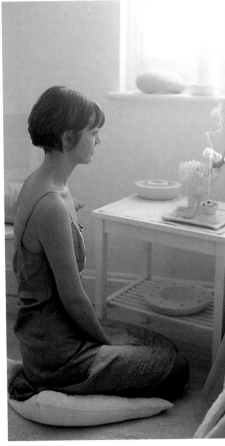

▲ Add a time for contemplation or prayer to your bedtime ritual.

49 lull yourself to sleep

At the end of a hectic day, soothing music can help you wind down in a pleasant way. Likewise, a blanket of neutral sound can help drown out the rest of the world, allowing deep relaxation.

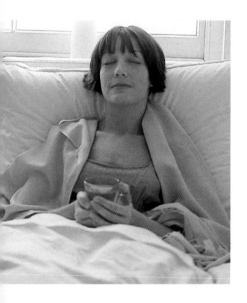

◀ Listen to your relaxing sounds as you sip a cup of herbal tea, or after you settle down.

Listening to pieces of classical music before bed may help you drift off to sleep. Music played on a single instrument, such as *Slow Pieces for Spanish Guitar* by Fernando Sor or piano pieces by Claude Debussy or Eric Satie, are good choices. New Age music is also ideal – often slow and repetitive, it brings a meditative state.

Make a tape or CD containing your favourite pieces of music. Avoid anything with a fast beat or sudden tempo changes. The more similar the pieces are in tempo and "feel", the more soporific will be the effect, as the repetition of similar notes will make your mind de-focus.

natural music
The sounds found in nature can have a hypnotic effect – very beneficial just before you go to bed. CDs are available containing sounds, such as the jungle, bird calls and whale songs. The sounds of the seashore are particularly relaxing and evocative.

calming noise
Some people find that white noise helps to curb the effects of environmental noise, such as background traffic or inconsiderate neighbours. Tune a radio to between stations, to where you will hear a hiss and turn the volume low. Alternatively, leave a fan running – its hum has a similar effect. If you find it comforting to hear people, leave on a talk radio station at a very low volume.

If you have a persistent **dream** try challenging it during the day. Light a **candle** to help you **focus** your thoughts, and consciously **relive** the dream. When you reach the disturbing part, take **control** and change the ending to a **happier** one.

index

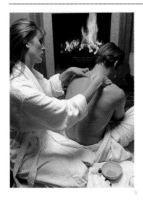

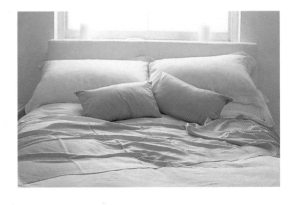

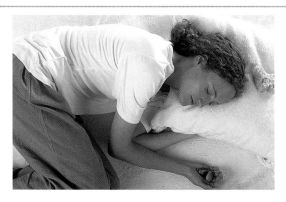

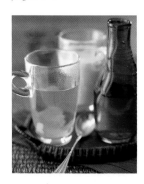

This edition is published by Lorenz Books

Lorenz Books is an imprint of Anness Publishing Ltd
Hermes House, 88–89 Blackfriars Road, London SE1 8HA
tel. 020 7401 2077; fax 020 7633 9499
www.lorenzbooks.com
info@anness.com
© Anness Publishing Ltd (2002)

Published in the USA by Lorenz Books,
Anness Publishing Inc.
27 West 20th Street, New York, NY 10011;
fax 212 807 6813

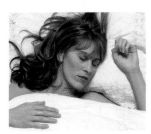

Published in Australia by Lorenz Books,
Anness Publishing Pty Ltd
Level 1, Rugby House, 12 Mount Street,
North Sydney, NSW 2060
tel. (02) 8920 8622; fax (02) 8920 8633

This edition distributed in the UK by Aurum
Press Ltd
25 Bedford Avenue, London WC1B 3AT
tel. 020 7637 3225; fax 020 7580 2469

This edition distributed in the USA by
National
Book Network
tel. 301 459 3366; fax 301 459 1705;
www.nbnbooks.com

This edition distributed in Canada by
General Publishing
tel. 416 445 3333; fax 416 445 5991;
www.genpub.com
This edition distributed in New Zealand by
David Bateman Ltd
tel. (09) 415 7664; fax (09) 415 8892

A CIP catalogue record for this book is
available from the British Library.

Publisher: Joanna Lorenz
Managing editor: Helen Sudell
Senior Editor: Joanne Rippin
Design: Jester Designs
Photography: Sue Atkinson, Martin Brigdale,
Nick Cole, John Freeman, Michelle Garrett,
Alistair Hughes, Andrea Jones, Don Last,
Lizzie Orme, Debbie Patterson,
Fiona Pragoff. .
Production controller: Joanna King
Editorial reader: Richard McGinley

1 3 5 7 9 10 8 6 4 2